Skills Worksheet
Directed Reading

Lesson: Facts About Drugs
DRUGS CHANGE THE MIND AND BODY

1. A _____ is any substance that changes how the mind or body works.

DRUGS ARE UNPREDICTABLE

2. List six factors that affect a person's reaction to drugs.

   _____
   _____
   _____
   _____
   _____
   _____

3. Besides unpredictable effects, what are two other risks from taking drugs?

   _____
   _____
   _____
   _____

Lesson: Medicine
WHAT IS A MEDICINE?

4. Define *medicine*.

   _____
   _____
   _____
   _____
   _____
   _____

Name _____ Class _____ Date _____

Directed Reading continued

DIFFERENT FORMS OF MEDICINE

5. Name five different forms medicines can take.

_____

_____

_____

_____

_____

OVER-THE-COUNTER MEDICINES

6. What are over-the-counter medicines?

_____

_____

7. Unexpected changes in the body or mind that are caused by medicines are called a _____.

PRESCRIPTION MEDICINES

8. What are prescription medicines?

_____

_____

READING A MEDICINE LABEL

_____ **9.** What information is found on a medicine label?
  a. how much to take
  b. how often to take it
  c. possible side effects
  d. All of the above

USING MEDICINES SAFELY

10. List three ways to use medicines safely.

_____

_____

_____

Copyright © by Holt, Rinehart and Winston. All rights reserved.

Decisions for Health — Understanding Drugs

Name _____ Class _____ Date _____

> **Directed Reading** continued

Lesson: Illegal Drugs
MARIJUANA

11. Which of the following is another name for marijuana?
   - **a.** pot
   - **b.** grass
   - **c.** weed
   - **d.** All of the above

12. What is a gateway drug?

_____

_____

_____

INHALANTS

_____**13.** Which of the following are chemical products that have strong fumes or odors?
   - **a.** anabolic steroids
   - **b.** inhalants
   - **c.** stimulants
   - **d.** depressants

ANABOLIC STEROIDS

14. Anabolic steroids can cause fast _____ gain and

muscle _____.

STIMULANTS AND DEPRESSANTS

15. What is the difference between a stimulant and a depressant?

_____

_____

OTHER ILLEGAL DRUGS

16. What are some effects of hallucinogens?

_____

_____

_____

Copyright © by Holt, Rinehart and Winston. All rights reserved.

Decisions for Health   3   Understanding Drugs

Name _____ Class _____ Date _____

Directed Reading *continued*

_____ **17.** Which of the following is a form of opiate?
  a. heroin
  b. marijuana
  c. cocaine
  d. sleeping pills

Lesson: Drug Abuse
MISUSE AND ABUSE

18. What is the difference between misuse and abuse of a drug?

_____
_____
_____
_____

THE COST OF ABUSING DRUGS

19. What risks and costs are involved with abusing drugs?

_____
_____
_____
_____

DRUG ABUSE AFFECTS DECISIONS

20. What types of decisions can drug abuse affect?

_____
_____

Lesson: Drug Addiction
BECOMING ADDICTED

_____ **21.** A condition in which a person needs more of a drug to feel the original effects of the drug is called
  a. withdrawal.
  b. dependence.
  c. tolerance.
  d. drug addiction.

Name _____ Class _____ Date _____

Directed Reading *continued*

22. What is withdrawal?

_____

_____

_____

23. The need to take a drug in order to feel normal is called _____.

24. The failure to control one's use of a drug is called _____.

RECOVERY
25. Why is withdrawal painful?

_____

_____

_____

Lesson: Refuse to Abuse
AVOIDING DRUG ENVIRONMENTS
26. What is one way to avoid social pressure to use drugs?

_____

_____

DRUG-FREE COPING
27. What is one drug-free way to cope with problems?

_____

_____

REFUSING OFFERS
28. List three different ways to refuse drugs.

_____

_____

_____

Decisions for Health — Understanding Drugs

Name _____ Class _____ Date _____

Skills Worksheet
Concept Mapping

Lesson: Facts About Drugs

Use the following terms to complete the concept map below: *mood, food in stomach, drugs, body weight, drug mix, amount of drug, drug allergies,* and *individual reaction.*

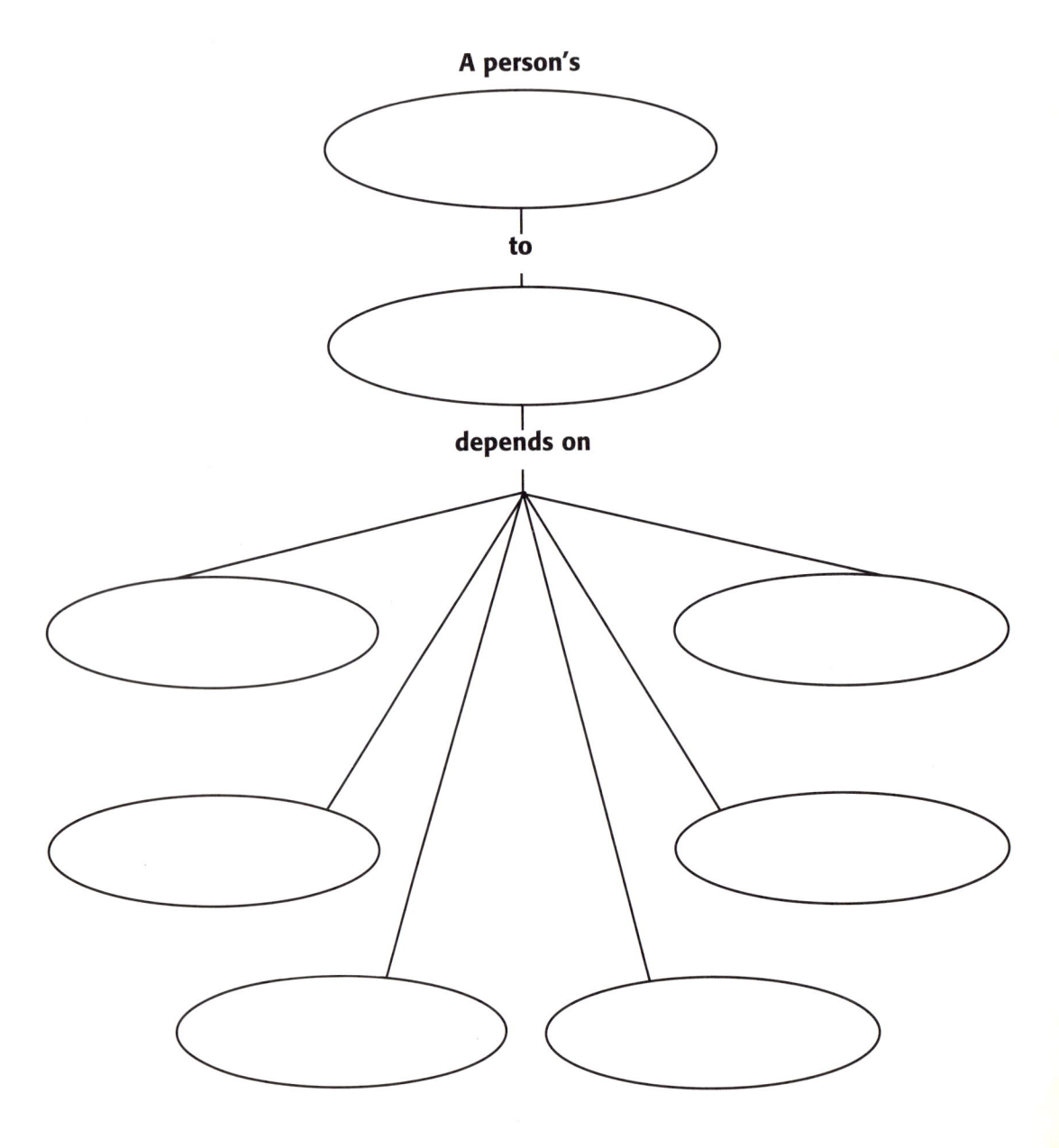

A person's

( )

to

( )

depends on

( ) ( ) ( ) ( ) ( ) ( )

Copyright © by Holt, Rinehart and Winston. All rights reserved.

Decisions for Health — Understanding Drugs

Name _____ Class _____ Date _____

Skills Worksheet
Concept Mapping

Lesson: Medicine

Use the following terms to create a concept map in the space below: *prescription medicine, medicine, over-the-counter medicine, side effects, prescription,* and *medicine label.*

Name _____ Class _____ Date _____

Skills Worksheet
Concept Review

Lesson: Facts About Drugs

_____ 1. Which factor can affect a person's reaction to a drug?
   a. the amount of drug he or she consumes
   b. how much he or she weighs
   c. how much food is in his or her stomach
   d. All of the above

2. Explain why food and water are not drugs.

_____
_____
_____

3. Can you predict how drugs will affect a person? Explain.

_____
_____
_____
_____

Lesson: Medicine

4. Define *medicine*.

_____
_____
_____

5. How can you use medicines safely?

_____
_____
_____

6. Explain the difference between over-the-counter and prescription medicines.

_____
_____
_____
_____

Name _____ Class _____ Date _____

Concept Review *continued*

7. Explain what side effects are.

_____

_____

_____

8. What information can be found on an OTC medicine label?

_____

_____

_____

9. List three ways to use medicines safely.

_____

_____

_____

_____

Lesson: Illegal Drugs

Match each definition with the correct term. Write the letter in the space provided.

_____ **10.** a drug that slows the body down

_____ **11.** a drug that speeds up body functions

_____ **12.** one of the most commonly used illegal drugs

_____ **13.** chemical product that has strong fumes or odors

_____ **14.** a drug that introduces people to drug use and increases the risk that they will try other drugs whose effects are stronger

_____ **15.** a drug that is abused to build muscle

_____ **16.** a drug that can make people see and hear things that do not exist

_____ **17.** a drug made from poppy flowers

a. marijuana
b. gateway drug
c. inhalant
d. anabolic steroid
e. stimulant
f. depressant
g. opiate
h. hallucinogen

Copyright © by Holt, Rinehart and Winston. All rights reserved.

Decisions for Health — Understanding Drugs

Name _____ Class _____ Date _____

> Concept Review *continued*

Lesson: Drug Abuse

18. Explain the difference between misuse and abuse.

_____
_____
_____

19. Name some social costs of abusing drugs.

_____
_____
_____

20. Explain how drug abuse affects decisions.

_____
_____
_____
_____

Lesson: Drug Addiction

Write the letter of the correct answer in the space provided.

_____ **21.** When a person cannot feel the original effects of a drug when taking the original amount of the drug, he or she has developed a
   a. drug addiction.
   b. withdrawal.
   c. tolerance.
   d. dependence.

_____ **22.** Needing a drug in order to feel normal is part of
   a. drug addiction.
   b. withdrawal.
   c. tolerance.
   d. dependence.

_____ **23.** The body's reaction to not having a drug that is usually present in the body is called
   a. drug addiction.
   b. withdrawal.
   c. tolerance.
   d. dependence.

Copyright © by Holt, Rinehart and Winston. All rights reserved.

Decisions for Health   Understanding Drugs

Name _____ Class _____ Date _____

Concept Review continued

_____ **24.** The failure to control one's use of a drug is called
  a. drug addiction.
  b. withdrawal.
  c. tolerance.
  d. dependence.

25. Explain why recovering from a drug addiction is difficult.

_____
_____
_____

Lesson: Refuse to Abuse

26. What can you do if someone invites you to a party where drugs may be used?

_____
_____
_____

27. How can you find ways to cope without drugs?

_____
_____
_____

28. Why is it important to think about ways to refuse drugs before they are offered to you?

_____
_____
_____

29. How can friends help you avoid drugs?

_____
_____
_____
_____

Name _____ Class _____ Date _____

Skills Worksheet
Refusal Skills

Lesson: Drug Abuse

Imagine you are the advice columnist for the school newspaper. Read the letter below and write a response to be published in the newspaper.

Dear Know-It-All,

I think one of my best friends may be abusing drugs. Her mom recently had surgery and was prescribed some really strong painkillers. One day, my friend had a headache and decided to try one of her mom's pills. She really liked the way it made her feel. My friend ended up taking the rest of the pills over the next few weeks. Now she's looking for a way to buy more of the pills without a prescription. She says she's desperate to get more pills. She asked me to look in my parents' medicine cabinet. What should I do?

Sincerely,

Worried

Name _____ Class _____ Date _____

Skills Worksheet
Refusal Skills

Lesson: Refuse to Abuse

Describe how you would use the following refusal skills to respond to the following scenario. Remember to be clear and choose your words carefully. Describe your body language as well as your words.

You are walking home from school with some of your friends. Bill lights up a joint and offers you a puff. Your other friends accept his offer. You hesitate, but Bill tells you that everyone smokes marijuana and that smoking marijuana is cool.

1. **Say no.** How would you say no to Bill?

   _____
   _____

2. **Offer an alternative.** What could you offer as an alternative?

   _____
   _____

3. **Stand your ground.** What would you do if Bill kept pressuring you to smoke?

   _____
   _____

4. **Walk away.** Describe how you would get out of the situation.

   _____
   _____

5. **Plan ahead.** What could you do to avoid this situation?

   _____
   _____
   _____
   _____

6. **Have a support system.** Who will stand by you when you are in this situation? How can you use these people as support when dealing with this situation?

   _____
   _____
   _____

Copyright © by Holt, Rinehart and Winston. All rights reserved.

Name _____ Class _____ Date _____

Skills Worksheet

Decision-Making Skills

Lesson: Illegal Drugs

Read the following situation. Then, follow the steps below to decide what you would do in this situation.

Your friend Chris invites you over to his house after school. When you get to his house, he asks you to go down into the basement with him. In the basement, he gets out a container of paint. Then, Chris starts to inhale the fumes from the paint. He encourages you to do it too. He says it will make you feel really good.

1. **Identify the problem.** What decision do you have to make?

   _____
   _____

2. **Consider your values.** What is important to you?

   _____
   _____

3. **List the options.** What possible actions could you take?

   _____
   _____
   _____

4. **Weigh the consequences.** List the pros and cons of each option.

   _____
   _____
   _____

5. **Decide and act.** Describe what you will do. Explain your decision.

   _____
   _____

6. **Evaluate your choice.** How do you feel about the action you took? Did you make a good decision? Would you take a different action if faced with the same scenario again?

   _____
   _____
   _____

Copyright © by Holt, Rinehart and Winston. All rights reserved.

Decisions for Health — Understanding Drugs

Name _____ Class _____ Date _____

Skills Worksheet

Decision-Making Skills

Lesson: Drug Abuse

Read the following story and then, use your knowledge of decision-making skills to write an ending to the story in the space below.

Eileen's friend Eva had been acting very strange lately. She was missing school a lot and sometimes she was mean to Eileen. Whenever Eileen saw Eva, Eva always asked to borrow money. Eileen couldn't figure out what was going on. Then one day, she caught Eva in the girls' bathroom taking some prescription drugs. Eileen asked her what they were, and Eva said her doctor prescribed them to her. Eileen was suspicious because she saw Eva taking many pills at once.

_____

_____

_____

_____

_____

_____

_____

_____

_____

_____

_____

_____

_____

_____

_____

_____

_____

_____

_____

_____

_____

_____

_____

Copyright © by Holt, Rinehart and Winston. All rights reserved.

Name _____ Class _____ Date _____

Skills Worksheet

Cross Disciplinary: Art

Lesson: Facts About Drugs

In a small group, create a poster for an anti-drug ad campaign. Imagine that your poster will become a billboard on the highway. Create something that is appealing and eye-catching. You may want to sketch your ideas in the space below.

Name _____ Class _____ Date _____

Skills Worksheet

Cross Disciplinary: Social Studies

Lesson: Drug Addiction

Interview a healthcare worker about drug addiction. You may want to ask the following questions and also make up some questions of your own.

1. What are the drugs that teens in this area are most likely to become addicted to?

   _____
   _____

2. What are some local resources teens can use to recover from drug addiction?

   _____
   _____

3. _____
   _____

4. _____
   _____
   _____

Write two paragraphs that summarize the interview.

_____
_____
_____
_____
_____
_____
_____
_____
_____
_____

Copyright © by Holt, Rinehart and Winston. All rights reserved.

Decisions for Health — Understanding Drugs

Name _____ Class _____ Date _____

Assessment

Quiz

Lesson: Facts About Drugs

Write the letter of the correct answer in the space provided.

_____ 1. Which of the following is a drug?
   a. food
   b. water
   c. cough syrup
   d. None of the above

_____ 2. Which of the following is an illegal drug?
   a. coffee
   b. marijuana
   c. cough syrup
   d. OTC pain relievers

_____ 3. Which of the following is NOT considered a drug?
   a. caffeinated tea
   b. alcohol
   c. food
   d. stimulants

_____ 4. Which factor affects how a person will react to a drug?
   a. how much food is in the stomach
   b. body weight
   c. what other drugs he or she is taking
   d. All of the above

_____ 5. Mixing one drug with another drug can
   a. change its effects.
   b. be good for you.
   c. help you solve your problems.
   d. None of the above

Copyright © by Holt, Rinehart and Winston. All rights reserved.

Decisions for Health — Understanding Drugs

Name _____ Class _____ Date _____

[Assessment]
Quiz

Lesson: Medicine

Write the letter of the correct answer in the space provided.

_____ 1. What is medicine used for?
   a. to cure disease
   b. to treat illness
   c. to prevent pain
   d. All of the above

_____ 2. Medicine that is inhaled
   a. reaches the blood very quickly.
   b. is slow to reach the blood.
   c. is never dangerous.
   d. is always good for you.

_____ 3. Which of the following is an example of an over-the-counter medicine?
   a. marijuana
   b. cough syrup
   c. steroids
   d. opiates

_____ 4. Which is an example of a prescription medicine?
   a. cough drops
   b. cocaine
   c. pain killer
   d. heroin

_____ 5. What does the label of a prescription medicine include that is NOT on the label of an OTC medicine?
   a. side effects
   b. how much to take
   c. how often to take it
   d. doctor's name

_____ 6. Which is NOT an example of using medicines safely?
   a. talking to your doctor about side effects
   b. being aware of allergies
   c. mixing with other drugs
   d. following directions

Copyright © by Holt, Rinehart and Winston. All rights reserved.
Decisions for Health   Understanding Drugs

Name _____ Class _____ Date _____

Assessment

Quiz

Lesson: Illegal Drugs

Match each definition with the correct term. Write the letter in the space provided.

_____ 1. a drug that slows the body down

_____ 2. a drug that speeds up body functions

_____ 3. a drug that is often smoked from a joint

_____ 4. a drug that introduces people to drug use and increases the risk that they will try stronger drugs

a. gateway drug

b. stimulant

c. depressant

d. marijuana

Write the letter of the correct answer in the space provided.

_____ 5. Which of the following is NOT an example of an illegal drug?
  a. coffee
  b. cocaine
  c. heroin
  d. marijuana

_____ 6. Which of the following is an effect of hallucinogens?
  a. seeing things that do not exist
  b. anxiety
  c. depression
  d. All of the above

_____ 7. Nail polish remover is an example of a(n)
  a. hallucinogen.
  b. inhalant.
  c. anabolic steroid.
  d. depressant.

_____ 8. Heroin is an example of a(n)
  a. opiate.
  b. inhalant.
  c. anabolic steroid.
  d. stimulant.

Copyright © by Holt, Rinehart and Winston. All rights reserved.

Decisions for Health — Understanding Drugs

Name _____ Class _____ Date _____

Assessment
Quiz

Lesson: Drug Abuse

Write the letter of the correct answer in the space provided.

_____ 1. The accidental incorrect use of a drug is called
   a. abuse.
   b. misuse.
   c. addiction.
   d. tolerance.

_____ 2. Purposefully using drugs incorrectly is called
   a. abuse.
   b. misuse.
   c. addiction.
   d. tolerance.

_____ 3. Which of the following is a risk involved in drug abuse?
   a. damage to physical health
   b. high financial costs
   c. loss of job
   d. All of the above

_____ 4. Drugs
   a. change the way a person's mind works.
   b. may influence a person's decisions about having sex.
   c. may influence how people decide to spend their time.
   d. All of the above

_____ 5. What can help you to make healthy decisions?
   a. smoking marijuana sometimes
   b. avoiding drugs
   c. relying on drugs to help you make decisions
   d. None of the above

Copyright © by Holt, Rinehart and Winston. All rights reserved.
Decisions for Health — Understanding Drugs

Name _____ Class _____ Date _____

Assessment

Quiz

Lesson: Drug Addiction

Write the letter of the correct answer in the space provided.

_____ 1. If a person is dependent on drugs, he or she has a
   a. withdrawal.
   b. drug addiction.
   c. tolerance.
   d. drug allergy.

_____ 2. When a person takes a drug many times, the body may develop a
   a. withdrawal.
   b. drug allergy.
   c. tolerance.
   d. prescription.

_____ 3. Craving a drug every day is a sign of
   a. peer pressure.
   b. side effects.
   c. tolerance.
   d. dependence.

_____ 4. Headaches, chills, and nausea can be symptoms of
   a. withdrawal.
   b. drug addiction.
   c. tolerance.
   d. dependence.

_____ 5. Withdrawal from an addiction
   a. is difficult.
   b. can be painful.
   c. can be dangerous.
   d. All of the above

Copyright © by Holt, Rinehart and Winston. All rights reserved.

Decisions for Health — Understanding Drugs

Name _____ Class _____ Date _____

Assessment
Quiz

Lesson: Refuse to Abuse
Write the letter of the correct answer in the space provided.

_____ 1. What is one way to avoid drugs?
   a. Go to parties where you know drugs will be used.
   b. Stay away from places where drugs are used.
   c. Make friends who use drugs.
   d. None of the above

_____ 2. If someone invites you to a party where drugs will be used, what should you do?
   a. Suggest going somewhere else.
   b. Stay home and use drugs.
   c. Go to the party.
   d. All of the above

_____ 3. Some people abuse drugs to
   a. cope.
   b. become healthier.
   c. look younger.
   d. None of the above

_____ 4. How can you refuse drugs?
   a. Say, "no, thanks".
   b. Suggest another idea.
   c. Walk away.
   d. All of the above

_____ 5. Drugs are
   a. the only way to have fun.
   b. dangerous and unpredictable.
   c. good for you.
   d. All of the above

Name _____ Class _____ Date _____

[Assessment]
Chapter Test

Understanding Drugs
USING VOCABULARY

Use the terms from the following list to complete the sentences below. A term may be used only once. Some terms will not be used.

drug	OTC medicine	prescription medicine	stimulant
hallucinogen	abuse	tolerance	withdrawal

1. A(n) _____ speeds up body functions.

2. You have developed _____ when you need more of a drug to feel its original effects.

3. A substance that changes how the mind or body works is called a(n) _____.

4. You can buy _____ without a doctor's written order.

5. Heroin is a type of _____.

6. Using an illegal drug is one kind of drug _____.

UNDERSTANDING CONCEPTS
Write the letter of the correct answer in the space provided.

_____ 7. A drug that is used to cure, treat, or prevent pain, disease, and illness is called a(n)
  a. anabolic steroid.
  b. depressant.
  c. medicine.
  d. inhalant.

_____ 8. A drug that slows the body down is called a(n)
  a. anabolic steroid.
  b. depressant.
  c. medicine.
  d. inhalant.

_____ 9. A drug that is abused to build muscles is called a(n)
  a. anabolic steroid.
  b. depressant.
  c. medicine.
  d. inhalant.

_____ 10. A chemical product with strong fumes is called a(n)
  a. anabolic steroid.
  b. depressant.
  c. medicine.
  d. inhalant.

Copyright © by Holt, Rinehart and Winston. All rights reserved.
Decisions for Health — Understanding Drugs

Name _____ Class _____ Date _____

Chapter Test *continued*

_____ 11. A doctor must give a written order for someone to purchase a(n)
  a. prescription medicine.   **c.** OTC medicine.
  b. inhalant.   **d.** hallucinogen.

_____ 12. A drug that increases the chance that someone will try stronger drugs is called a
  a. depressant.   **c.** hallucinogen.
  b. gateway drug.   **d.** stimulant.

_____ 13. Accidentally using a drug incorrectly is called
  a. tolerance.   **c.** misuse.
  b. dependence.   **d.** abuse.

_____ 14. The body's reaction to not having a drug that is usually present in the body is called
  a. dependence.   **c.** tolerance.
  b. abuse.   **d.** withdrawal.

CRITICAL THINKING

15. Explain why it is important to read medicine labels carefully.

_____

_____

_____

16. Describe three ways to ensure that you use medicines safely.

_____

_____

_____

17. What are the effects of long-term marijuana use?

_____

_____

_____

18. What are the dangers of abusing inhalants?

_____

_____

_____

_____

Copyright © by Holt, Rinehart and Winston. All rights reserved.
Decisions for Health   Understanding Drugs

Name _____ Class _____ Date _____

Chapter Test *continued*

19. Explain how withdrawal from an addiction makes it difficult for a person to stop using a drug.

_____

_____

_____

_____

_____

_____

_____

20. Nicole's friend Stacy is pressuring her to smoke marijuana. Stacy tells Nicole that marijuana always makes people feel really good. Explain what factors may affect how Nicole's body would react to the marijuana. Then, explain whether it is true that marijuana always makes people feel really good.

_____

_____

_____

_____

_____

_____

21. Ginger is at a party where some of her friends are using drugs. They keep asking her to join in. Describe three ways that Ginger could refuse the drugs.

_____

_____

_____

_____

_____

_____

Name _____ Class _____ Date _____

Chapter Test *continued*

INTERPRETING GRAPHICS

Examine the diagram below, and answer the questions that follow.

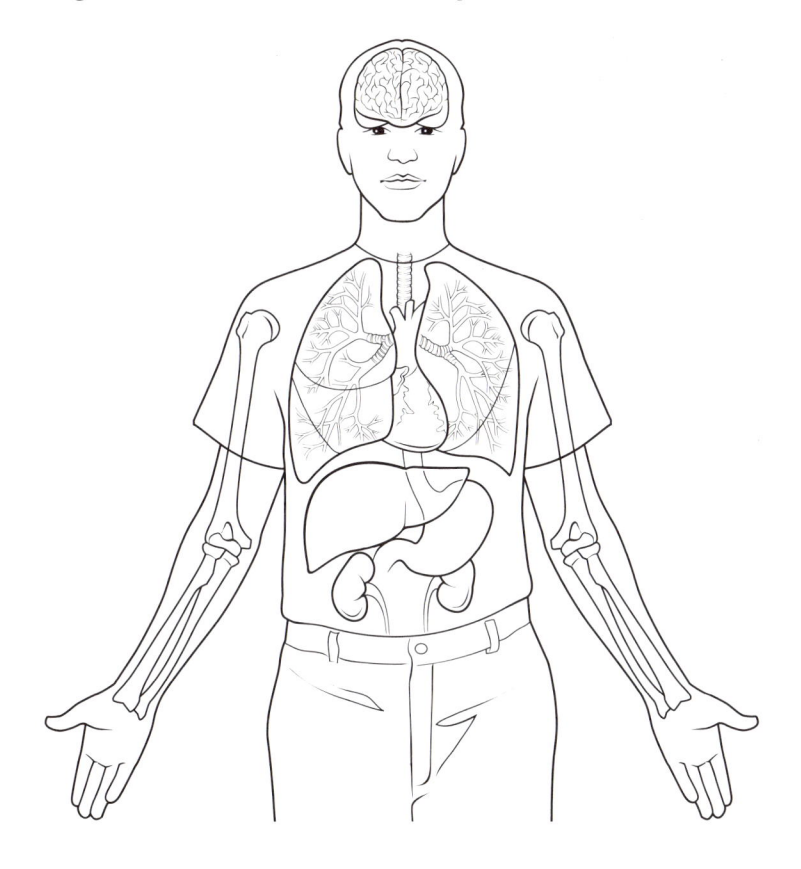

22. What can happen to your ability to breathe when you abuse inhalants?

_____
_____
_____
_____
_____

23. How can inhalant abuse harm internal organs?

_____
_____
_____
_____
_____
_____
_____

Name _____ Class _____ Date _____

> Assessment

Performance-Based Assessment

Understanding the Dangers of Drugs

INTRODUCTION

You've read about the different types of drugs and the effects of drug abuse. Now you will have a chance to help others understand the dangers of drug abuse.

OBJECTIVE

- Keep in mind that your teacher will be observing and grading your in-class behavior as well as your written responses. In particular, your teacher will be noting your ability to follow the given procedures, how well you follow classroom safety guidelines, and your methods and reasoning in solving problems.
- Try not to let what others are doing influence your work. Remember that a problem often has several acceptable solutions.
- Do not talk to other students unless you are working in a group. Talk only to members of your group and try not to disturb other students.
- Use only the materials provided.

SAFETY CAUTIONS

Use caution when using the scissors and stapler.

MATERIALS AND EQUIPMENT

- pen or pencil
- notepad
- several sheets of unlined paper
- scissors
- stapler
- markers

PROCEDURE

1. Work with one or two other students. Imagine that you are the school nurse. You want to warn students about the dangers of drugs. Create a short presentation and a brochure that discusses different types of drugs and their possible effects.
2. Use the unlined paper, scissors, stapler, and markers to create your brochure. It should be easy to read and appealing to look at.
3. Write and rehearse your presentation. You can base your presentation on the information in your brochure.
4. Give your presentation to the entire class. Listen carefully to the presentations of others.

Copyright © by Holt, Rinehart and Winston. All rights reserved.

Decisions for Health — Understanding Drugs

Name _____ Class _____ Date _____

Performance-Based Assessment *continued*

ANALYSIS

Answer the following questions in the space provided. Support your answers by explaining your reasoning.

1. Do you think people your age would read a brochure about the dangers of drug abuse if they were given one? Explain.

   _____
   _____
   _____
   _____
   _____
   _____
   _____
   _____

2. What information do you think is the best deterrent against drug abuse for people your age?

   _____
   _____
   _____
   _____
   _____
   _____
   _____

3. What is the best way to approach people your age about the dangers of drug abuse? Is it more effective to be approached by a peer or by an adult, such as a school nurse or parent, about the subject? Explain your answer.

   _____
   _____
   _____
   _____
   _____
   _____
   _____

Name _____ Class _____ Date _____

Activity

Datasheet for In-Text Activity

Drug and Chemical Safety

1. Examine empty boxes and containers from household chemical products and medicines provided by your teacher.
2. Label the table below with columns for
    (1) the name of each product
    (2) chemicals in each product
    (3) dangers of each chemical or product
    (4) first-aid responses for exposure to each product
3. Fill in the table by using the information on the labels of the chemical product containers.

Copyright © by Holt, Rinehart and Winston. All rights reserved.

Decisions for Health — Understanding Drugs

Name _____ Class _____ Date _____

Datasheet for In-Text Activity *continued*

ANALYSIS

1. What are some dangers of these common household products? Are these dangers similar to the dangers of using illegal drugs?

   _____
   _____
   _____
   _____
   _____
   _____
   _____

2. What should you do if you accidentally breathe, swallow, or touch these products?

   _____
   _____
   _____
   _____
   _____
   _____
   _____

Name _____ Class _____ Date _____

Activity

Life Skills: Being a Wise Consumer

Lesson: Medicine
THE IMPORTANCE OF MEDICINE LABELS

Read the following situation. Then, answer the questions.

You have a really bad headache, so you get an over-the-counter pain medicine. You read the label and take two pills. Two hours later, your head is still hurting. You look at the medicine label again. It says to take one to two pills every four to six hours. Your head is really hurting.

1. What should you do before taking any over-the-counter medicine?

   _____
   _____
   _____
   _____

2. Should you take another pill before the recommended time? Explain your answer.

   _____
   _____
   _____
   _____

3. Why is it important to carefully read the labels on over-the-counter drugs?

   _____
   _____
   _____
   _____

4. If your headache gets worse and does not go away, what can you do?

   _____
   _____
   _____
   _____

Copyright © by Holt, Rinehart and Winston. All rights reserved.

Decisions for Health   **Understanding Drugs**

Name _____ Class _____ Date _____

Activity
Life Skills: Coping

Lesson: Drug Addiction
DEALING WITH STRESS

Read the following situation. Then, answer the questions.

You are having a really bad week. You failed a test and you got in a huge fight with your best friend. Another friend, Ryan, notices you are down. He says he has just the solution to your problems. He offers you a marijuana joint. Ryan tells you it will make you relax, feel good, and forget all of your problems. He tells you he smokes it every day.

1. Why might you want to take the joint?

   _____
   _____
   _____
   _____

2. Should you take the joint to feel better?

   _____
   _____
   _____
   _____

3. What could happen if you do decide to smoke the joint?

   _____
   _____
   _____
   _____

4. List some other ways you can cope with your problems besides turning to drugs.

   _____
   _____
   _____
   _____

Copyright © by Holt, Rinehart and Winston. All rights reserved.

Name _____ Class _____ Date _____

Activity
Enrichment Activity

Lesson: Facts About Drugs

Survey 25 students at your school. Ask each student to:

- name some common illegal drugs.
- describe what he or she knows about the negative effects of drug use.

Now make a list of the five most common illegal drugs that were named. In general, do you think the people you surveyed are well-educated about drugs? What were some drugs not mentioned? What were some harmful side effects not mentioned? Write two or three paragraphs to summarize your findings.

Lesson: Medicine

Use a separate sheet of paper to write a story in which a student has a health problem, but is not sure whether it requires medicine. The story should include ideas for how to try feeling better without using medicine.

Lesson: Illegal Drugs

Many young people believe marijuana and inhalants are "safe" drugs. Use the library or government websites to research the possible effects of marijuana and inhalant abuse. After your research, ask yourself if they are "safe" drugs. Use a separate sheet of paper to write several paragraphs that summarize your findings.

Name _____ Class _____ Date _____

Enrichment Activity *continued*

Lesson: Drug Abuse

Go to the library and research the laws regarding drug abuse in your state. Find out what happens to first-time drug offenders and to repeat drug offenders. Use a separate sheet of paper to write a report on your findings. Tell whether you think the penalties for drug abuse are too harsh or not harsh enough. Justify your response.

Lesson: Drug Addiction

Do research on the various support programs for people with drug addictions. Find out how hospitals and rehabilitation centers help people recover from addiction. Prepare an oral presentation that summarizes your research. On a separate sheet of paper, record your sources and data.

Lesson: Refuse to Abuse

Produce a video that demonstrates how to refuse drugs. Assume the video will be used to teach younger students to say no to drugs. Make sure your video covers the following topics:

- Different ways to say no
- Providing alternatives
- Social activities that do not involve drugs

Name _____ Class _____ Date _____

Activity
Health Inventory

Resisting Peer Pressure

Here is a checklist about drugs. Put a check next to each statement that describes you.

_____ 1. I know that drugs are unpredictable.

_____ 2. I read the labels on over-the-counter medications carefully before taking them.

_____ 3. I read the labels on prescription medications carefully before taking them.

_____ 4. I avoid situations in which I might be offered illegal drugs.

_____ 5. I know that using inhalants can have serious consequences for my health and can even cause death.

_____ 6. I know that using anabolic steroids is not a healthy way to build muscle.

_____ 7. I know I risk making unhealthy decisions if I use drugs.

_____ 8. I know the signs of drug addiction and know where to go for help if I think someone has a problem.

_____ 9. I can think of many fun things to do that don't involve drugs.

_____ 10. I know that the best way to avoid drug addiction is to never start abusing drugs.

Give yourself one point for each checkmark. Write your score here _____.

7–10 points: Excellent—You know the facts about drugs.
4–6 points: Good—You know some of the facts, but you should know more.
Under 4 points: Poor—You would benefit from learning more about drugs.

Name _____ Class _____ Date _____

Activity

Health Behavior Contract

Understanding Drugs

My Goals: I, _____, will accomplish one or more of the following goals:

I will stay drug free.

I will know where to get help if a friend or I ever need help dealing with a drug problem.

I will use refusal skills if drugs are offered to me.

Other: _____

_____

My Reasons: By staying drug free, using refusal skills, and being prepared to deal with drug-related problems, I will be promoting my health and safety. Being drug free will allow me to pursue my interests, maintain relationships, and reach other goals.

Other: _____

_____

My Values: Personal values that will help me meet my goals are

_____

_____

_____

My Plan: The actions I will take to meet my goals are

_____

_____

_____

Evaluation: I will use my Health Journal to keep a log of actions I took to fulfill this contract. After 1 month, I will evaluate my goals. I will adjust my plan if my goals are not being met. If my goals are being met, I will consider setting additional goals.

Signed _____

Date _____

Copyright © by Holt, Rinehart and Winston. All rights reserved.

Decisions for Health — Understanding Drugs

Name _____ Class _____ Date _____

Activity
At-Home Activity

Understanding Drugs

With a parent, look at some of the over-the-counter medicines you have in your house. Read and discuss their labels.

1. What information is on the labels?

   _____
   _____
   _____
   _____

2. Why is it important to check the expiration date before using a medicine?

   _____
   _____
   _____
   _____

3. List some of the possible side effects you found listed on the medicine labels.

   _____
   _____
   _____
   _____

4. Besides reading the label, what else should you do before taking any medicine?

   _____
   _____
   _____
   _____

The signatures below verify that our discussion has take place.

_____   _____
Student Signature   Class Period

_____   _____
Parent or Guardian Signature   DateActivity

Copyright © by Holt, Rinehart and Winston. All rights reserved.
Decisions for Health   Understanding Drugs

Name _____ Class _____ Date _____

Activity

Actividad En Casa

El entendimiento de las drogas

Con su padre/madre/tutor, mire algunos de los medicamentos disponibles sin receta que hay en su casa. Lea y discuta las etiquetas.

1. ¿Qué información da la etiqueta?

_____
_____
_____

2. ¿Por qué es importante hacer caso de la fecha de caducidad antes de tomar un medicamento?

_____
_____
_____

3. Haga una lista de algunos de los efectos secundarios descritos en las etiquetas.

_____
_____
_____

4. Además de leer la etiqueta, ¿qué más se debe hacer antes de tomar un medicamento?

_____
_____
_____

Las firmas verifican que discutimos esta actividad juntos.

_____   _____
Firma de Estudiante   Período de Clase(la Salud)

_____   _____
Firma de Padre/Madre/Tutor   Fecha

TEACHER RESOURCE PAGE

Parent Letter

Understanding Drugs

Dear Parent/Guardian,

In the years to come, your child will be making decisions that impact his or her physical, emotional, and social health. The purpose of this Health Education class is to provide students with the knowledge and resources they need to make responsible and well-informed decisions about their health. As the course progresses, students will be asked to explore their values, opinions, and beliefs about health. It is important that students receive mature guidance in the classroom and at home as they address these issues.

In the next few weeks, your son or daughter's Health Education class will focus on the subject of drugs. Your child's ability to make good decisions about drug use will influence not only how long he or she lives, but also the quality of his or her life years from now. The chapter will introduce strategies for resisting pressure to use drugs.

Other topics covered in this chapter include over-the-counter and prescription medication as well as drug addiction.

You can actively support your child's progress in Health by communicating with him or her about the topics covered in this course. To aid this communication, I have included a worksheet for you to complete with your child. This worksheet is entitled *Understanding Drugs*, and it provides guidance for an in-depth discussion. Your signature at the end of this material will verify that this home interaction has taken place.

Thank you in advance for your time, cooperation, and support.

Sincerely,

_____

Health Teacher

Carta a los Padras/al Tutor

El entendimiento de las drogas

Estimado(s) Padres/Tutor:

En el futuro, su hijo/a va a hacer decisiones que influyan en su salud física, emocional y social. El motivo fundamental de la clase de Salud es proporcionarles a los estudiantes los conocimientos y recursos precisos para hacer responsables decisiones bien informadas en cuanto a su salud. Durante el año académico, los alumnos tendrán que revisar sus valores, opiniones y creencias sobre la salud. Es importante que, al confrontar estos asuntos, los jóvenes reciban informes y consejos de adultos tanto en el aula de clases como en casa.

En las próximas semanas, la clase de Salud se enfocará en el tema de las drogas. La capacidad de hacer buenas decisions sobre el uso de las drogas va a influir tanto en cuántos años su hijo/a viva como la calidad de su vida en el futuro. El capítulo va a presentar estrategias para resistir la initimidación para usar drogas.

Otros asuntos tratados en este capítulo son los medicamentos con y sin receta y la adicción a las drogas.

Ud. puede ayudar a su hijo/a en esta clase por hablar con él o ella sobre los temas que estudie. Para facilitar esta comunicación le mando una hoja de trabajo, El entendimiento de las drogas, para completar con su hijo/a. Esta hoja da motivo por una discusión más a fondo. Su firma en la hoja verifica que Uds. discutieron esta actividad juntos.

Gracias anticipadas por su tiempo, cooperación y apoyo.

Atentamente,

_____

Maestro/a de Salud

TEACHER RESOURCE PAGE

Assessment
Performance-Based Assessment

Understanding the Dangers of Drugs

Teacher's Notes
INTRODUCTION

Students will create a brochure and deliver a presentation about the dangers of drug abuse.

TIME REQUIRED One 45-minute class period.

Students will need 20 minutes to create their brochures and prepare their presentations and 25 minutes to give their presentations.

PBA RATINGS Easy ←— 1 2 3 4 —→ Hard
  Teacher Prep—1
  Student Set-Up—1
  Concept Level—2
  Clean Up—1

ADVANCE PREPARATION

Obtain enough unlined paper, scissors, staplers, and markers for each group of students.

SAFETY CAUTIONS

Remind students to use caution when using the scissors and stapler.

PERFORMANCE

At the end of the test, students should turn in the following item:
- Completed brochure

EVALUATION

The following is a recommended breakdown for evaluating student performance:
  30% Completion of brochure
  40% Understanding of the effects of drug abuse
  30% Delivery of presentation

TEACHER RESOURCE PAGE

Answer Key

Directed Reading

LESSON: FACTS ABOUT DRUGS
1. drug
2. weight, mood, food, mixing, amount, allergies
3. Taking drugs can put relationships and lives at risk. It can also affect a person's responsibilities.

LESSON: MEDICINE
4. A medicine is a drug that is used to cure, treat, or prevent pain, disease, and illness.
5. pill, liquid, syrup, cream, spray
6. medicines that can be bought without a doctor's written order
7. side effects
8. medicines that can be bought only with a written order from a doctor
9. d
10. Follow directions; never mix drugs; be aware of allergies.

LESSON: ILLEGAL DRUGS
11. d
12. A gateway drug is a drug that introduces people to drug use, increasing the risk that they will try stronger drugs.
13. b
14. weight, growth
15. Stimulants are drugs that speed up body functions. Depressants are drugs that slow the body down.
16. They can make people see and hear things that do not exist. They can cause people to do dangerous things. They also cause anxiety and depression.
17. a

LESSON: DRUG ABUSE
18. Misuse is the accidental incorrect use of a drug. Abuse is the purposeful incorrect use of drugs or the use of an illegal drug.
19. damage to physical health; losing friends, families, and jobs; inability to concentrate on responsibilities; high financial costs
20. decisions about having sex, decisions about how to spend your time

LESSON: DRUG ADDICTION
21. c
22. Withdrawal is the body's reaction to not having a drug that is usually present in the body.
23. dependence
24. drug addiction
25. because the body has been used to large amounts of a drug

LESSON: REFUSE TO ABUSE
26. to stay away from places where they are used
27. talking to a friend or trusted adult
28. Say "no, thanks"; give a reason; walk away.

Concept Mapping

LESSON: FACTS ABOUT DRUGS
A person's *individual reaction* to *drugs* depends on *mood, food in stomach, body weight, drug mix, amount of drug*, and *drug allergies*.

LESSON: MEDICINE
Answers may vary. Sample answer: *Medicines* include *prescription medicine*, which can be taken only with a *prescription*, and *over-the-counter medicines*, both of which can have *side effects* that should be listed on the *medicine label*.

Concept Review

LESSON: FACTS ABOUT DRUGS
1. d
2. because the body needs them every day in order to function properly
3. No; Different people can react differently to the same drug. The same person can react differently to the same drug at different times.

TEACHER RESOURCE PAGE

LESSON: MEDICINE
4. a drug that is used to cure, treat, or prevent pain, disease, and illness
5. Follow instructions from a doctor or a medicine's label.
6. OTC medicines can be bought without a doctor's written order. Prescription medicines can be bought only with a prescription.
7. unexpected changes in the body or mind that are caused by medicines
8. how much to take, how often to take it, when it's too old to use, possible side effects
9. Follow directions; never mix drugs; be aware of allergies

LESSON: ILLEGAL DRUGS
10. f
11. e
12. a
13. c
14. b
15. d
16. h
17. g

LESSON: DRUG ABUSE
18. Misuse is the accidental incorrect use of a drug. Abuse is the purposeful incorrect use of drugs or the use of an illegal drug.
19. People who abuse drugs can harm or destroy relationships. They can also lose the ability to concentrate, causing them to lose their jobs or do poorly in school.
20. Drugs change the way your mind works, which makes it difficult to make healthy decisions.

LESSON: DRUG ADDICTION
21. c
22. d
23. b
24. a
25. Addicted people who stop using drugs go through withdrawal, which can be painful and dangerous.

LESSON: REFUSE TO ABUSE
26. Do not go; suggest going somewhere else.
27. Talk to a friend or trusted adult, speak to a counselor, see a doctor, call a teen hotline.
28. If you ever face that situation, you will know what to do.
29. Friends who share your ideas about drugs can set examples of how to refuse drugs. They can support you when you act on your decisions about drugs. They can also enjoy drug-free activities with you.

Refusal Skills

LESSON: DRUG ABUSE
Answers may vary. Sample answer: Dear Worried, Your friend does have a drug problem. You are right to be worried. You should refuse to help her get more drugs. If you feel comfortable, try talking to your friend about her problem. You might be able to convince her to seek help. If she is unresponsive, you should talk to a trusted adult, such as a parent or school counselor. Drug addiction is serious and without help your friend could experience many negative health effects, or even die. Sincerely, Know-It All

LESSON: REFUSE TO ABUSE
Answers may vary. Accept all reasonable answers. Sample answers:
1. I would tell Bill I am not interested in smoking marijuana.
2. I could ask if everyone wants to go rollerblading instead.
3. I would tell Bill that smoking pot is illegal and dangerous.
4. I would tell my friends I have to run an errand and walk home alone.
5. Answers may vary. Sample answer: I could avoid situations where I think drugs might be used.
6. Answers may vary. Sample answer: I have friends who do not do drugs. They will stand by my decision not to do drugs.

TEACHER RESOURCE PAGE

Decision-Making Skills

LESSON: ILLEGAL DRUGS
Answers may vary. Accept all reasonable answers. Sample answers:
1. I have to decide if I will inhale the paint fumes or not.
2. My health is important to me.
3. I could inhale the fumes, I could ask Chris to stop, or I could go home.
4. If I inhale the fumes, I may harm my body. If I ask Chris to stop, he may get mad at me. Or, he might like it if I suggest another activity. If I just go home, he may get mad at me, but I will be protecting my health.
5. I will ask Chris to stop. If he does not, I will go home.
6. I am happy with my decision. I know it was the best thing for me. I have other friends who like to have fun without drugs.

LESSON: DRUG ABUSE
Answers may vary. Sample answer: Eileen kept pestering Eva about what she saw in the bathroom. Eva finally admitted to her that the pills did not come from the doctor. She had first gotten some from a friend and then started looking for other places to buy the pills. Eileen was very upset, but she wanted to help Eva. She asked Eva to talk to the school counselor about her problem.

Cross Disciplinary: Art

LESSON: FACTS ABOUT DRUGS
Students' posters may vary. They should attempt to convince people to stay away from drugs and should be appealing and eye-catching.

Cross Disciplinary: Social Studies

LESSON: DRUG ADDICTION
Students should write two paragraphs that summarize their interviews with a healthcare worker about drug abuse.

Quizzes

LESSON: FACTS ABOUT DRUGS
1. c
2. b
3. c
4. d
5. a

LESSON: MEDICINE
1. d
2. a
3. b
4. c
5. d
6. c

LESSON: ILLEGAL DRUGS
1. c
2. b
3. d
4. a
5. a
6. d
7. b
8. a

LESSON: DRUG ABUSE
1. b
2. a
3. d
4. d
5. b

LESSON: DRUG ADDICTION
1. b
2. c
3. d
4. a
5. d

LESSON: REFUSE TO ABUSE
1. b
2. a
3. a
4. d
5. b

Chapter Test

1. stimulant
2. tolerance
3. drug
4. OTC medicines

Copyright © by Holt, Rinehart and Winston. All rights reserved.

Decisions for Health — Understanding Drugs

TEACHER RESOURCE PAGE

5. opiate
6. abuse
7. c
8. b
9. a
10. d
11. a
12. b
13. c
14. d
15. Answers may vary. Sample answer: Reading labels can help you use medicines safely. They tell how much to take, how often to take it, and when a medicine is too old to use. They also warn of any possible side effects.
16. Answers may vary. Sample answer: Follow directions from doctors on medicine labels. Never mix drugs unless a doctor tells you to. Be aware of any allergies you may have.
17. Answers may vary. Sample answer: It can damage the lungs and cause problems similar to those caused by smoking tobacco, such as cancer.
18. Answers may vary. Sample answer: They can make the heart stop beating and keep a person from getting enough air. They can cause brain damage, hearing loss, and damage to the kidneys, liver, and bones. They can also lead to death.
19. Answers may vary. Sample answer: People who try to quit may start using drugs again to avoid the painful symptoms of withdrawal.
20. Answers may vary. Sample answer: Nicole's body weight and mood can affect her reaction to the drug. The amount of food Nicole has eaten is also a factor. If Nicole is taking any other drugs, the effects of the marijuana can be altered. The amount of the drug Nicole uses as well as any allergies she may have will also affect her body's reaction to the drug. With so many factors involved, it is impossible to say that marijuana always makes people feel really good.
21. Answers may vary. Sample answer: She could say "no, thanks." She could also give a reason for not using the drugs, saying it's illegal. She could also leave the party to get away from the situation.
22. Answers may vary. Sample answer: Your lungs can fill with chemicals and your airways can become blocked.
23. Answers may vary. Sample answer: It can cause brain damage, hearing loss, bone deterioration, heart attack, liver damage, and kidney damage.

Performance-Based Assessment

1. Answers may vary. Sample answer: Yes, because it is an interesting topic and many of us have already been in situations with drugs.
2. Answers may vary. Sample answer: telling us the possible harmful effects and that drug abuse can result in death
3. Answers may vary. Sample answer: Many of us watch TV everyday, so TV commercials are an effective tool. It's more effective to be approached by a peer because we can relate to each other better.

Datasheet for In-Text Activity

1. Answers may vary. Sample answers: poisoning, asphyxiation, death, nausea; Yes, these dangers are similar to the dangers of using illegal drugs.
2. Answers may vary. Sample answers: Wash your body, call Poison Control, go to the emergency room.

Life Skills: Being a Wise Consumer

LESSON: MEDICINE
1. Answers may vary. Sample answer: Read the label
2. Answers may vary. Sample answer: No, there could be harmful side effects if you take too much.

TEACHER RESOURCE PAGE

3. Answers may vary. Sample answer: so you can know how much to take, how often to take it, and the possible side effects
4. Answers may vary. Sample answer: Call the doctor.

Life Skills: Coping

LESSON: DRUG ADDICTION
1. Answers may vary. Sample answer: I might want to take it because I am feeling so lousy.
2. Answers may vary. Sample answer: No, I should not take the joint and it would not help me feel better.
3. Answers may vary. Sample answer: I could become addicted and turn to drugs whenever I have a problem.
4. Answers may vary. Sample answers: Talk to a friend or adult about my problems or do something fun to get mind off of my problems without using drugs.

Enrichment Activity

LESSON: FACTS ABOUT DRUGS
Students should list the five most common illegal drugs mentioned in their surveys and write several paragraphs to summarize their findings.

LESSON: MEDICINE
Students' stories should show informed decision making about treating the health problem and include ideas for trying to feel better without using medicine.

LESSON: ILLEGAL DRUGS
Students should write several paragraphs that summarize their findings on marijuana and inhalants.

Enrichment Activity

LESSON: DRUG ABUSE
Students' reports may vary, but they should make an argument about whether or not they think the penalties for drug abuse are too harsh.

LESSON: DRUG ADDICTION
Students should prepare an oral presentation that describes the various support programs and rehabilitation centers available to help people recover from drug addiction.

LESSON: REFUSE TO ABUSE
Students should make a video that demonstrates to younger kids how to refuse drugs. Their videos should cover different ways to say no, providing alternatives, and social activities that do not involve drugs.

Health Inventory
Student responses may vary. This worksheet can be used to start a discussion on drug misuse and abuse.

Health Behavior Contract
Accept all reasonable responses.

At-Home Activity
Answers may vary. Sample answers:
1. how much to take, how often to take it, expiration date, possible side effects
2. If the medication is too old, it may not work properly or it may become bad for you.
3. Student responses may vary based on the medicines they looked at.
4. Get permission from a parent.